Raynaud's Syndrome

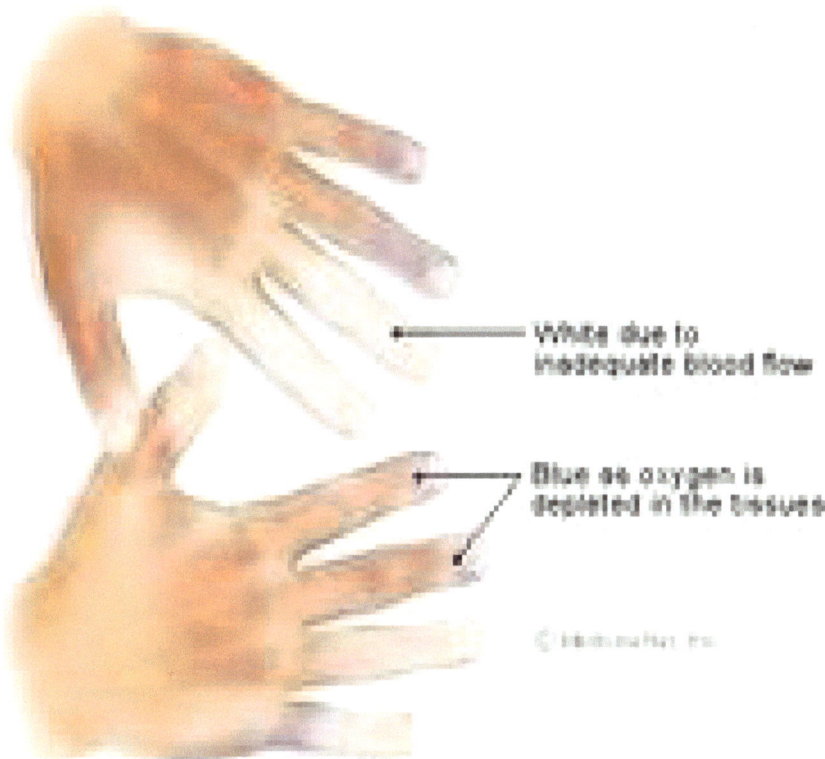

Table of Contents

1. **Title of book**   Page 1
2. **Table of contents**   Page 2
3. **Dedication page**   Page 3
4. **Actual book**   Pgs. 4-43
5. **Book synopsis**   Page 44
6. **Author's biography**   Page 45

Dedication Page

This book is dedicated to my beloved mother, Sharon

Introduction to Raynaud's Syndrome

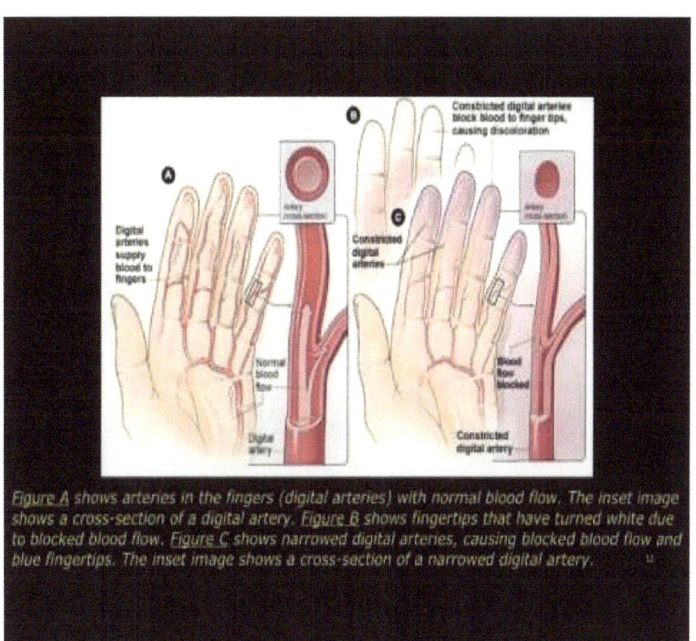

Courtesy of edexitvideo

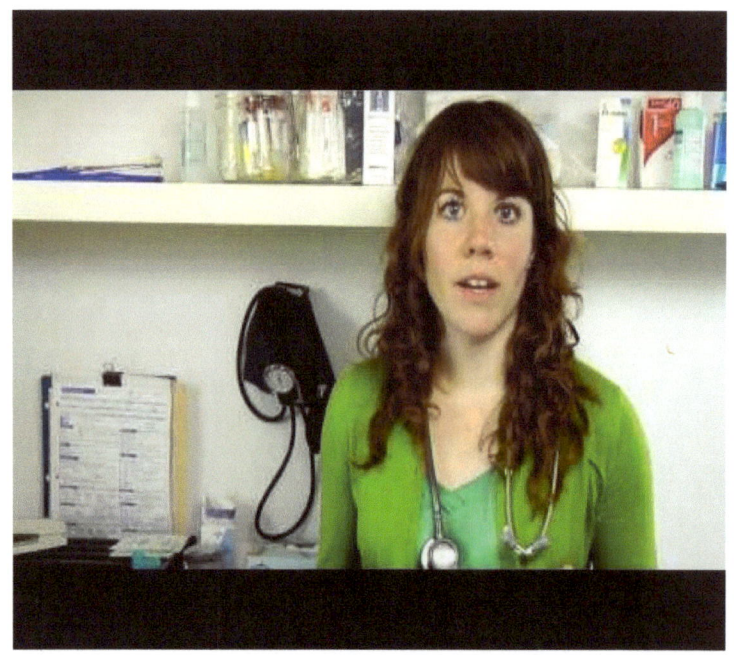

Courtesy of eHowhealth

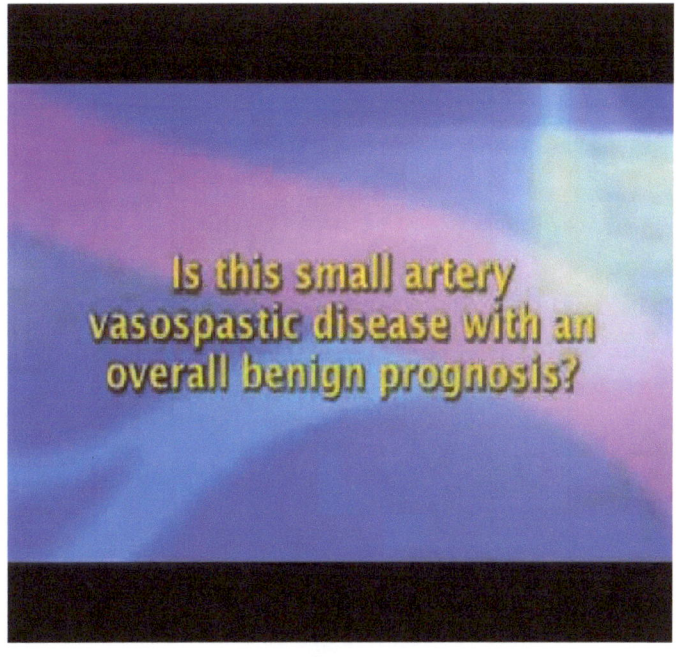

Courtesy of SVS Vascular

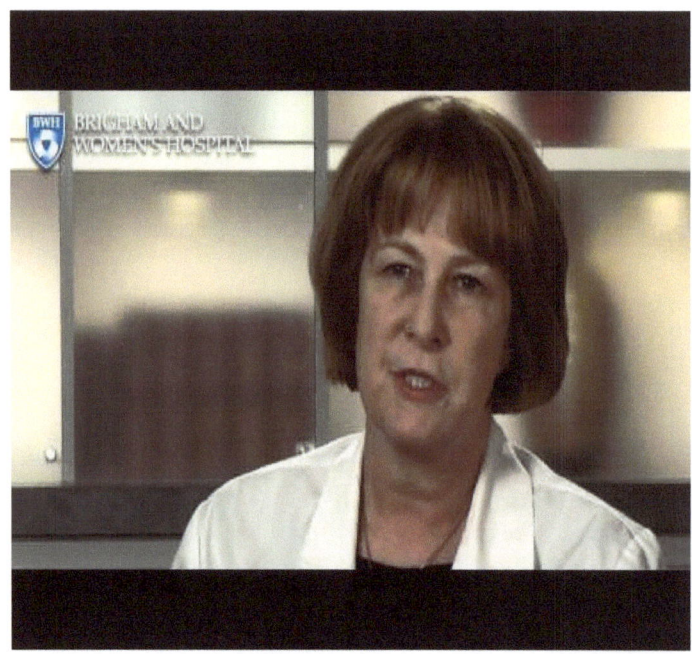

Courtesy of Brigham and Women's Hospital

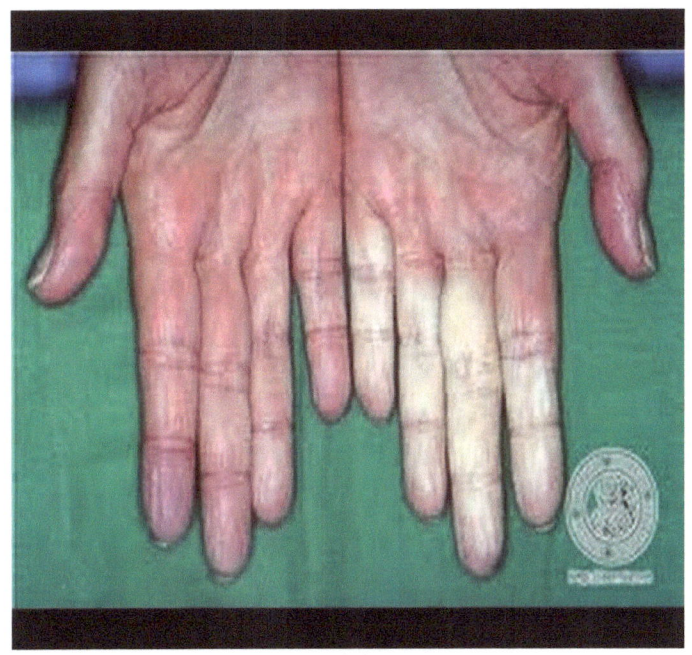

Courtesy of Chef Mama Rosa (Vegan)

Raynaud's phenomenon and/or Raynaud's syndrome is defined as the reduced and excessive blood supply in response to emotional stress and/or the cold temperatures.
In the field of modern medicine, this disease may cause discoloration of the digits (fingers and toes) and other places on occasion.

Raynaud's syndrome can also cause a person's fingernails and toe nails to become brittle with longitudinal ridges.

Maurice Raynaud (1834-1881) was a French physician for which the disease was actually named.

The Raynaud phenomenon is believed to cause vasospasms that will cause a decrease in the supply of blood flow to any and all of the respective regions.

If the anomaly's cause is idiopathic, it will be called Raynaud's disease, also called primary Raynaud's.
If the anomaly is caused by a secondary condition such as Scleroderma, it will be correctly referred to as Raynaud's phenomenon, also called secondary Raynaud's.

Raynaud's phenomenon has been known to contain pathophysiology which included hyper activation of the sympathetic nervous system.
This can cause extreme vasoconstriction of the peripheral blood vessels.
This can lead to tissue hypoxia.
If a patient or someone you know has recurrent or chronic cases of Raynaud's phenomenon and/or Raynaud's syndrome, atrophy of the skin, muscle atrophy, as well as subcutaneous tissue atrophy may result.

In some documented rare cases of patients, ischemic gangrene and/or ulceration may result as well.

Signs and Symptoms of Raynaud's phenomenon or Raynaud's Syndrome

Raynaud's syndrome may cause paleness or discoloration, numbness, cold sensations and/or affected extremity pain.
This can make a person that has yet to be diagnosed to become distressed and sometimes even obstructive.
If a person actually has Raynaud's syndrome and is placed into a cold climate for a long period of time it may become extremely dangerous for the individual.

Some unique signs may be as follows:

- If the digits(fingers and toes), earlobes as well as the nose become exposed to cold temperatures the supply of blood could be reduced
- The skin may become pallor(white or pale) as well as numb and cold if a person with Raynaud's is exposed to cold climate conditions
- Cyanosis could result as well if the oxygen is depleted for some odd reason and the person's skin will turn blue

➢ Some of the Raynaud's episodes only happen on occasion but generally once the area affected is warmed and the blood supply returns, the color of the skin may appear rubor (turned red), then the skin will return to its normal color but it may be followed by painful "pins and needles", swelling or even a tingling sensation could develop.

- Everyone needs to know if they have a mild case of Raynaud's or a more severe case of the disease
- Everyone should also take notice that a reactive hyperemias may actually cause some of the symptoms if the areas are deprived from blood flow

- ➢ In pregnancy patients, the above aforementioned sign may disappear because it owes this to increased surface blood flow
- ➢ Breastfeeding mothers may also obtain Raynaud's syndrome
- ➢ If the breastfeeding mother actually does have Raynaud's syndrome, her nipples may

- Become extremely painful and turn pallor(white or pale)
- In one medical study, a calcium channel blocker and/or vasodilator called Nifedipine was recommended to the breastfeeding mothers so that it may increase the supply of blood to the extremities which notably relieved some of the breast pain in one small medical study group

Some of the main causes of Raynaud's phenomenon or Raynaud's Syndrome

If a person has the primary Raynaud's syndrome (Primary Raynaud's) their symptoms may be idiopathic.

Idiopathic symptoms actually means that they are simply caused by themselves and are not caused by any other disease.

Sometimes, the Primary Raynaud's disease may be referred as "being allergic to the cold".

This disease generally develops when women get into their teenage years or early adulthood.

Primary Raynaud's disease has been thought to be partly hereditary, however, the medical community has not yet identified any genes that are actually connected to this disease.

Smoking may also increase the intensity and frequency of each Raynaud attack and hormonal components are also a contributing factor.

Caffeine can also worsen each attack.

Most sufferers are more likely to have angina and severe migraines.

If a person has Secondary Raynaud's Syndrome then it can be caused by a multitude of conditions.

Secondary Raynaud's has several associations:

- Connective Tissue Disorders
- Cold agglutinin disease
- Ehler's Danlos syndrome
- Mixed connective tissue disease
- Polymyositis

- Sjogren's syndrome
- Dermatomyositis
- Scleroderma
- Rheumatoid arthritis
- Systemic lupus erythematosus

Eating Disorders

Anorexia Nervosa

- **Obstructive Disorders**

- **Subclavian aneurysms**

- **Thoracic outlet syndrome**

- **Takayasu's arteritis**

- **Buerger's disease**

- **Atherosclerosis**

- **Drugs**

- **Ergotamine**

- **Sulfasalazine**

- **Anthrax vaccines**

- **Ciclosporin**

- **Beta-blockers**

- **Cytotoxic drugs**

- **Bromocriptine**

- **Stimulant medications**

- **OTC medications also**

Some jobs or occupations may also cause Raynaud's Syndrome

Here are some of the occupations below:

- ✓ Drilling and weed whacking may suffer from vibration white finger

- ✓ Mercury and vinyl chloride exposure

- ✓ Cold exposure

There are also several other contributing factors that may cause Raynaud's Syndrome

Other contributing factors could be as follows:

- Auto accidents
- Physical trauma
- Hypothyroidism
- Lyme disease
- Malignancy
- Cryoglobulinemia
- Chronic fatigue syndrome
- Carpal tunnel syndrome
- Reflex sympathetic dystrophy

- **Multiple sclerosis**
- **Magnesium deficiency**
- **Erythromelalgia**

Raynaud's can herald all of these diseases for periods as long as twenty years in some case studies.

If this happens, Crest Syndrome can occur.

Secondary Raynaud's patients may also have some symptoms that can be related to some other underlying disease. Scleroderma patients usually gets Raynaud's syndrome as its initial symptoms.

Scleroderma is a skin and joint disease and it occurs about 70% of the time.

If a person just has symptoms in one hand or foot, this is called Unilateral Raynaud's.

This is a very uncommon form of this disease and it generally always plays secondary to a local or regional vascular disease.

Unilateral Raynaud's usually progresses to affect other limbs within several years.

Diagnosis of Raynaud's Syndrome

There is a three-step process in diagnosing Raynaud's phenomenon:

1) Ask screening questions
2) Assess color changes
3) Calculate the disease score

It is very important that medical professions distinguish the difference between Raynaud's disease (Primary Raynaud's) and Raynaud's phenomenon (Secondary Raynaud's).

The medical professional needs to do as follows:

1) Take a careful medical history
2) Perform digital artery pressure
3) Doppler ultrasound
4) Full blood count
5) Blood tests
6) Thyroid function testing
7) Autoantibody screenings and others
8) Nail fold vasculature

Conclusions

Raynaud's phenomenon (secondary Raynaud's) is managed by treating all of the underlying causes and by avoiding emotional and environmental stress, cold temperatures, vibrations, avoiding smoking, repetitive motions and sympathomimetic drugs. Surgery and Low level laser therapy can also help a person with this disease.

Raynaud's phenomenon and/or Raynaud's syndrome is a disease that causes excessive reduced blood flow in a person's fingers, toes, and other areas occasionally. This is usually brought on by emotional stress and colder temperatures. This self-help book discusses some of the signs and symptoms, some of the causes, gives some ways as to how medical professions may diagnose the disease and how a person may be able to actually manage this disease. If you suspect that you or someone you know may have this disease, please discuss this medical condition with your physician the next time you have an appointment with your healthcare professional.

Misty Lynn Wesley is a diversified career professional in the medical, legal, fashion, and insurance industries. She is an avid blogger for Examiner.com and she has written articles for CBS Local out of St. Paul, MN. She has also published four books with Publish America and several with Create Space in order to keep the book prices more affordable for her readers. Her love of the medical profession was her true inspiration in writing this medical self-help book on Raynaud's Syndrome and she hopes that you enjoy the book. God bless!!!